Apple Cider Vinegar Miracle Handbook: The Ultimate Health Guide to Silky Hair, Weight Loss, and Glowing Skin!

How to Use Apple Cider Vinegar to Prevent Candida, Allergies, Acne, Acid Reflux, Heart Burn and Arthritis Plus find more Benefits.

Disclaimer

Table of Contents

Apple Cider Vinegar Miracle Handbook: The Ultimate Health Guide to Silky Hair, Weight Loss, and Glowing Skin! 1

Disclaimer 2

Summary 7

Introduction 8

1. How to make Apple Cider Vinegar at Home? 9

    Ingredients 9

    Directions 9

    Storage Directions 10

2. Benefits of Apple Cider Vinegar 11

3. The Best Way to Consume Apple Cider Vinegar 12

    Mixing with Water 12

    Dressing 12

    Drinking with Lemon 12

    Consuming with Raw Vegetables and Fruits 12

4. Apple Cider Vinegar- All-In-One Cure 13

    4.1. Apple Cider Vinegar for Weight Loss 14

        How Apple Cider Vinegar Works? 14

        Best Way to Consume 14

        Is Apple Cider Vinegar Effective in Weight Loss? 15

    4.2. Apple Cider Vinegar for Skin Care 16

        Apple Cider Vinegar Remedies for Glowing Skin 16

        Apple Cider Vinegar for Acne Control 17

    4.3. Apple Cider Vinegar for Acid Reflux 18

        Apple Cider Vinegar and Water 18

        Apple Cider Vinegar and Honey 18

        Apple Cider Vinegar with Salads 19

    4.4. Apple Cider Vinegar for Allergies 20

How to take Apple Cider Vinegar? 20

4.5. Apple Cider Vinegar for Silky Hair 21

How to Wash Hair with Apple Cider Vinegar? 21

4.6. Apple Cider Vinegar for Diabetes 22

How Apple Cider Vinegar Controls Diabetes 22

Ways to Consume Apple Cider vinegar for Diabetes 22

4.7. Apple Cider Vinegar for Yeast Infection 24

How to Use Apple Cider Vinegar for Yeast Infection 24

4.8. Apple Cider Vinegar for Arthritis 26

Apple Cider Vinegar Cure for Arthritis 26

4.9. Apple Cider Vinegar for High Cholesterol 28

How to Consume? 28

4.10. Apple Cider Vinegar for High Blood Pressure 29

Apple Cider Vinegar with Honey Remedy 29

Apple Cider Vinegar with Salads 29

Apple Cider Vinegar with Cayenne Pepper 30

5. Uses of Apple Cider Vinegar 31

5.1. Toner 31

Apple Cider Vinegar Toner 31

5.2. Mouth Wash 32

Apple Cider Vinegar Mouth Wash 32

5.3. Face Mask 32

Apple Cider Vinegar Face Mask 33

5.4. Bath Solution 33

Apple Cider Vinegar Bath Solutions 33

5.5. Wart Removal 34

Wart Removal Remedy 34

5.6. Veins Treatment 35

Apple Cider Vinegar Veins Cure 35

5.7. Deodorant 36

5.8. Sun burn Remedy 36

5.9. Stomach Issues 37

5.10. Stuffy Nose 37

5.11. Hiccups 38

5.12. Swelling/Sore Throat 38

5.13. Leg Cramps 39

5.14. Exhaustion 39

5.15. Bad Breath 40

5.16. Skin Fungus 40

5.17. Low Blood Pressure 41

5.18. Age Spots 41

6. Easy Homemade Apple Cider Vinegar Recipes **42**

6.1. Lunch 42

Apple Cider Vinegar with Fried Chicken and Onion 42

Apple Cider Vinegar Roasted Vegetables 43

6.2. Dinner 44

Baked Chicken with Apple Cider Vinegar 44

Apple Cider Vinegar glazed Pork Chops 45

6.3. Drinks 46

Apple Cider Vinegar Detox 46

Apple Cider Vinegar Cocktail 47

6.4. Salads 48

Apple Cider Vinegar Harvest Salad 48

Apple Cider Vinegar Mushroom Salad 49

6.5. Desserts 50

Apple Cider Vinegar Sponge Cake 50

Apple Cider Vinegar Ice Pops 51

6.6. Dips and dressings 52

Apple Cider Vinegar Strawberry Dressing 52

Apple Cider Vinegar Honey Dressing 53

Final Words **54**

Summary

Contrary to the normal perception that vinegars are only used for cooking, apple cider vinegar has a number of health benefits which you will be amazed to know about. If you are looking for home remedies to prevent Candida, allergies, acne, acid reflux, heart burn and arthritis, then you have come to the right place. This eBook includes a number of apple cider vinegar remedies which are not only effective for treating allergies but they can also serve the purpose of beauty enhancement products.

Along with revealing the use of apple cider vinegar as a health tonic, the book also contains some healthy and easy to prepare recipes which will facilitate regular and adequate consumption of apple cider vinegar. With an inclusive compilation of apple cider vinegar recipes, the eBook unveils the use of apple cider vinegar as mouth wash, deodorant and many more!
If you are looking for an ultimate health guide to weight loss, spotless skin and healthy hair, then keep reading.

Introduction

As the name implies, apple cider vinegar is a product formed after the fermentation of apple cider. Unlike apple juice, cider does not undergo the process of filtration and therefore contains fruit pulp. Like all other types of vinegar, apple cider vinegar also goes through several stages of fermentation. During the first stage of fermentation, fructose in apple pulp is turned into alcohol, after reacting with yeast. Cider alcohol is further fermented to produce vinegar.

Apple cider vinegar contains the nutrition of apple along with lactic and citric acids. This is the reason that ACV is not only used for cooking but modern studies have also singled it out as an effective tonic for weight loss and other diseases.

1. How to make Apple Cider Vinegar at Home?

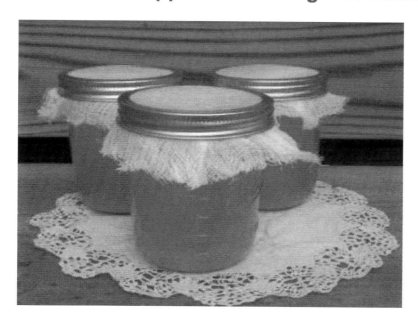

There are a number of manufacturers of apple cider vinegar, but looking for a quality brand can be a little frustrating when you have a number of options to choose from. Here is a simple recipe which can help you in making apple cider vinegar at home.

Ingredients

Note: These ingredients will produce 1 gallon cider vinegar.

10 apples

Cinnamon (optional), 1 tbsp

Allspice (optional), 1 tbsp

White Sugar, ¾ cup

Water

Directions

Wash apples thoroughly to remove debris. Cut each apple into four pieces and crush them together to form apple pulp. Wrap the pulp in cheesecloth and squeeze it hard into a container. You can add a pinch of yeast if you want to accelerate the process of fermentation, but it is recommended to go with natural fermentation.

Leave the container uncovered, but place it a dark place to avoid direct exposure of sunlight. Maintain a moderate temperature (60°F-80°F). Stir the juice ever few days to remove any molds. Afte5 a few days bubbles will start to form indicating that the process of fermentation has been completed.

Filter the vinegar using a fine pours cloth or cheesecloth and pour it into a saucepan for pasteurization. Heat the vinegar to 140°F. Make sure that the heating temperature does not exceed 160ºF. You can use a thermometer to keep a track of temperature. Pasteurization helps in keeping the vinegar in excellent condition for several days and prevents further fermentation. Cool the vinegar till it reaches normal room temperature and store it into a clean container.

Storage Directions

Don't use a metal container for storing ACV. Vinegar has the tendency to corrode metals and rust particles can cause serious stomach infection. Moreover make sure that the container is air tight and completely dried.

2. Benefits of Apple Cider Vinegar

Apple cider vinegar is not only used in salads and dressings, but it can also replace a number of antibiotics. Among the list of health issues ACV can address, the most prominent one is weight loss. Unlike other types of vinegars, ACV does not only contain a combination of different acids but it also contains a number of vitamins and minerals which facilitate healthy weight loss.

Many people associate ACV with cooking and weight loss but this amazing organic vinegar can also serve the purpose of an inclusive beauty care product. You might have noticed that apple is used in most skin care products. ACV combines the nutrition of apple and bacteria fighting characteristics of vinegar to cure serious skin infections.

A number of people rely on diet pills and fat burners to control cholesterol levels, but apple cider vinegar is one of the most effective home remedies to control cholesterol and reduce the risk of cardiovascular diseases.

3. The Best Way to Consume Apple Cider Vinegar

Although modern studies suggest that you can reap countless health benefits by consuming apple cider vinegar on daily basis, a number of people avoid it due to its tanginess. However, there are a number of ways through which you can change the taste of apple cider vinegar and consume it regularly. Some of the simplest ways are:

Mixing with Water

The simplest way to dilute the taste of apple cider vinegar is to mix it with distilled water. All you have to do is take a glass of water and add two tablespoons of good quality apple cider vinegar to it. You can also add a pinch of sugar or honey to sweeten the solution. Consume this health tonic thrice a day and stay healthy.

Dressing

Another way to make the most of this organic health tonic is to use it in dressings and dips. Apple cider vinegar dressings are east to make and can be stored for months. You can use these dressings with salads or you can also use apple cider vinegar in dessert toppings.

Drinking with Lemon

Adding 2 tablespoons of apple cider vinegar and lemon juice to a glass of hot water, acts as a very effective weight loss remedy. As lemon is also an effective fat killer, the combination of apple cider vinegar and lemon juice allows you to lose weight quickly. The mixture also serves the purpose of anti-toxin tonic. You can also add cinnamon in this mixture. Adding herbs to the mixture of water and apple cider vinegar doubles the effectiveness of this health tonic.

Consuming with Raw Vegetables and Fruits

You can use apple cider vinegar to season raw fruits and vegetables. Consuming apple cider vinegar with fresh vegetables not only keeps the daily calorie intake low, it also facilitates proper functioning of the heart by keeping the cholesterol level low.

You can find some amazing apple cider vinegar dinner, lunch, dessert, salad and dressing recipes in this eBook.

4. Apple Cider Vinegar- All-In-One Cure

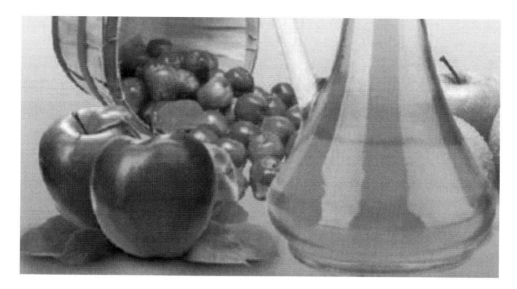

Modern studies have confirmed the fact that apple cider vinegar is an amazing health tonic which is not only effective in weight loss but it can also cure diseases like diabetes, abrupt blood pressure and even arthritis. ACV contains a wide rand of vitamins which can help in keeping the skin glowing and minerals like sulfur, iron, and potassium ensure proper functioning and development of all vital organs.

Modern studies have unveiled countless health benefits of ACV. Some of these benefits are:

- Weight loss
- Skin care
- Acid reflux treatment
- Allergies prevention
- Silky hair
- Diabetes control
- Yeast infection treatment
- Cholesterol control
- Stable blood pressure

Let us see these health benefits of consuming apple cider vinegar in detail:

4.1. Apple Cider Vinegar for Weight Loss

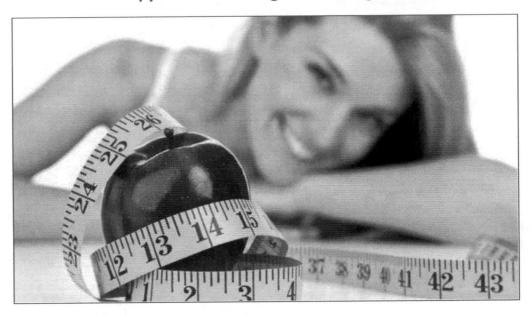

A number of people rely on diet pills and appetite suppressants for losing weight. Although these products help in weight loss by accelerating metabolism, there are a number of long term side effects of diet pills. However, ACV offers a natural way to prevent fat accumulation without any side effects. While a number of people claim that ACV is effective in weight loss, they don't have adequate knowledge about weight loss action of ACV.

How Apple Cider Vinegar Works?

A number of theories suggest that ACV works in the similar manner as weight loss pills. As ACV contains a mixture of organic acids which accelerate metabolism and enzymes in vinegar suppress appetite. Moreover, ACV also contains a wide range of vitamins which help in keeping the body healthy.

Modern studies have confirmed that apple cider vinegar is one of the healthiest weight loss tonics. The organic product helps in suppressing appetite by controlling blood sucrose levels. Moreover, apple cider vinegar also triggers insulin secretion which helps in preventing fat accumulation.

It is very important for weight loss to avoid eating during meals. Scientists suggest that apple cider vinegar can help you in feeling fuller by controlling blood sugar.

Best Way to Consume

In order to make the most of ACV for weight loss, health experts recommend taking two teaspoons of ACV before each meal. However if you don't like the taste of ACV, you can consume it with a glass of water. Diet experts also suggest that dissolving 2 teaspoons of raw honey and ACV in a glass of water and consuming it before each meal helps in suppressing appetite and cutting down extra fact.

Is Apple Cider Vinegar Effective in Weight Loss?

According to experimental studies, ACV consumption does not only help in weight loss but it also helps in keeping the body healthy. It is estimated that, with no change in the diet plan, consuming 2 teaspoons of ACV before each meal can help in losing 15 pounds in a year. However, with strict dieting daily consumption of ACV can result in 2 pounds weight loss per week.

4.2. Apple Cider Vinegar for Skin Care

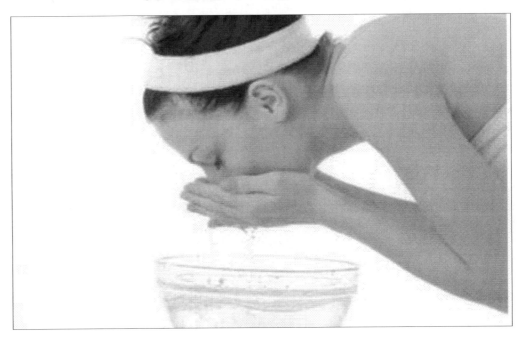

The concept of using apple cider vinegar as a beauty care product is not new. The use of this organic product for skin care can be traced back to the 19th century when Romans used a number of dried plants and vinegar for cosmetic purposes.

Apple cider vinegar keeps the skin healthy by facilitating proper blood circulation in skin capillaries. Moreover, the product also acts an antiseptic and enhances immunity against viruses and bacteria which cause skin infection. ACV also keeps the skin clear by removing dust particle from skin pores and absorbing oily deposits. As apple cider vinegar is acidic in nature, it helps in maintaining the neutral pH of skin.

Apple Cider Vinegar Remedies for Glowing Skin

There are a number of types of apple cider vinegar, but for cosmetic purposes white ACV is the most suitable option. ACV when mixed with dried plants can do wonders to skin. Here are some of the tested remedies, which can help you in keeping skin fresh and glowing:

- Take 3 oz. of *elder flower* and 2 oz. of *calendula* and crush them together. Add 2-3 pints of white apple cider vinegar and leave the mixture to macerate for 2 weeks.
- Take 1 oz. of *rose petals, lime flowers* and *lavender* and crush them together. Add 2-3 pints of white apple cider vinegar and leave the mixture to macerate for 2-3 weeks.
- Take 0.4 teaspoon of *rosewood oil* and 0.6 teaspoon of *rosemary* and *lavender oil* and mix them together. Then add 17-18 fl. Oz of white apple cider vinegar and mix all the ingredients thoroughly. Add 2 tablespoons of glycerin in the end.

It is recommended to store these mixtures in an air tight and screw top jar. To use, add 1 teaspoon of mixture to a bowl of water and wash your face. These remedies have no side effects.

Apple Cider Vinegar for Acne Control

Following apple cider vinegar remedies are effective in acne control:

- Take half cup of white apple cider vinegar, one cup of *orange blossom water* and quarter cup of *honey*. Mix all the ingredients well and wash your face with the mixture before sleeping. You can also add 2-3 drops of lavender oil for fragrance. For quick results, apply the mixture to your face and leave it overnight. The remedy is also very effective in getting rid of blemishes and dark spots. You can also use *green tea* solution instead of orange blossom water.
- Another tested apple cider vinegar remedy for acne control is to add *green tea* to hot water and allow the solution to cool. Add 1/3 cup of distilled water and white apple cider vinegar to green tea solution. Apply the mixture to your skin before sleeping and leave it on overnight. Rinse it off with cold water in the morning.

4.3. Apple Cider Vinegar for Acid Reflux

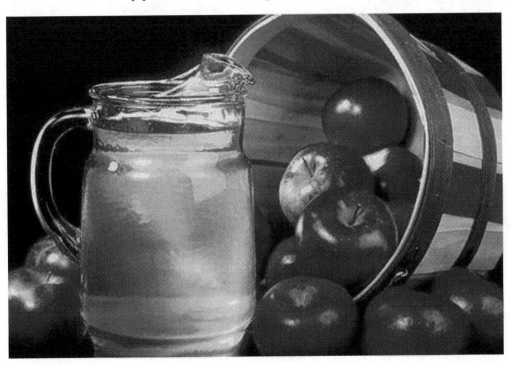

Acids secretion in stomach helps in food digestion. But when glands start secreting excessive amount of acids, a person is said to suffer from acid reflux. Acid reflux, as the name implies, is the condition when stomach acids start entering esophageal tract. These acids cause irritation in esophagus, stomach ache and nausea.

Apple cider vinegar can help you cure the problem of acid reflux without any side effects. Although apple cider vinegar contains high percentage of acetic acid, it reduces the pH levels of stomach acid. The mixture of weak acids in ACV reacts with strong stomach acids and corrects the pH balance in stomach. With reduced ph stomach produces lesser amount of acids. Unlike medicines, apple cider vinegar does not only cure acid reflux but it also ensures proper functioning of stomach.

Apple Cider Vinegar and Water

This is the simplest apple cider vinegar remedy for acid reflux. Add 1-2 tablespoons of good quality apple cider vinegar to a glass of water. Drink the mixture during meals. If the vinegar is too strong, you van increase the amount of water to dilute the solution.

Apple Cider Vinegar and Honey

Another remedy for neutralizing stomach acids is to mix 2 table spoons of honey and white apple cider vinegar together and consume it before meals. Raw honey is rich in potassium and helps in correcting the pH of stomach acids. The mixture also helps in preventing indigestion.

Apple Cider Vinegar with Salads

In order to consume apple cider vinegar on daily basis, it is recommended to add small amounts of ACV to salads or pickles. To make the most of ACV, consume it with raw vegetable salads.

You can also add make apple cider vinegar side dishes like bean salads. Boil and drain 1.5 cups of beans. Add finely chopped onion and 2 tablespoons of white apple cider vinegar to beans.

4.4. Apple Cider Vinegar for Allergies

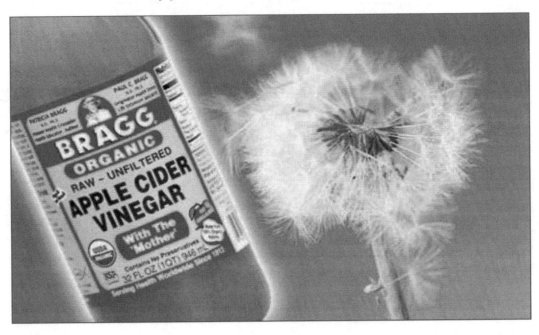

Allergies are caused due to weak immune systems. According to an estimate by the Food and Drug Administration (FDA), millions of people all over the world suffer from seasonal allergies. Common allergens include pollen grains and dust particles. Although there are a number of medicines for seasonal allergies, they cannot strengthen the immune system against allergens. However, apple cider vinegar is not only effective in curing allergies, but it is also strengthens immunity.

How to take Apple Cider Vinegar?

There are a number of ways to consume apple cider vinegar on a daily basis. Some of the simplest remedies are:

- Add 1 teaspoon of white apple cider vinegar to 0.5 liter of distilled water. Consume the mixture thrice a day.
- Another way to take apple cider vinegar for allergies is to add 2-3 drops of apple cider vinegar to 1 tablespoon of raw honey.

4.5. Apple Cider Vinegar for Silky Hair

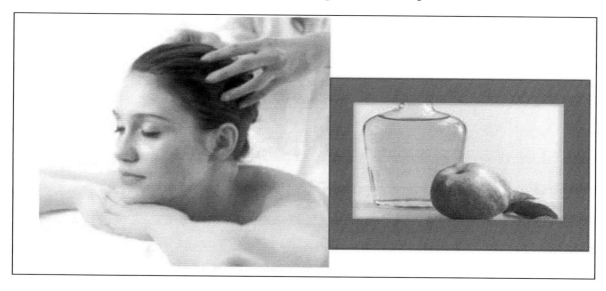

Rinsing hair regularly with good quality apple cider vinegar is a simple way to get rid of dandruff and oily hair. The cleansing action of vinegar helps in removing small particles of dust which ordinary shampoo fails to do. Although apple cider vinegar is considered as one of the oldest natural beauty care product, a number of people don't know the exact procedure of washing hair with apple cider vinegar. Here is a simple procedure which can help you in getting shiny and silky hair, the remedy is also effective in repairing split ends.

How to Wash Hair with Apple Cider Vinegar?

To prepare apple cider vinegar hair wash you will need ½ cup of water and ½ cup of white apple cider vinegar. The proportion is suitable for short to medium hair but if you have extra long hair you should take 1 cup of water and vinegar. Mix them together in a large bowl. Wash your hair with a regular shampoo. Apply apple cider vinegar mixture to wet hair and massage gently. Leave it on scalp for 5-10 minutes and then rinse your hair thoroughly. The formula is also effective in facilitating hair growth. For quick results, it is recommended to rinse hair with apple cider vinegar twice a week.

4.6. Apple Cider Vinegar for Diabetes

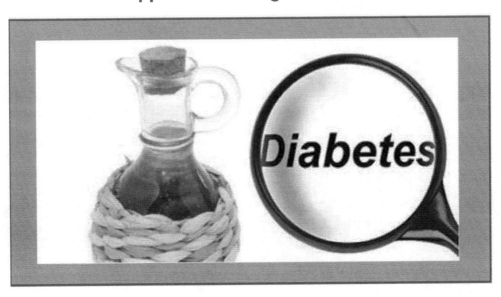

How Apple Cider Vinegar Controls Diabetes

Although people have been using apple cider vinegar to cure diabetes for years, many people don't have knowledge about how this organic tonic controls diabetes. Before 2004, it was thought that apple cider vinegar works in a similar manner as Precose (drug) and controls insulin secretion by slowing down the absorption of sugar into the blood.

But recent studies show that apple cider vinegar does not only slow sugar absorption but it can also lower postprandial glucose levels. It means that apple cider vinegar can naturally increase insulin sensitivity, which most of the insulin controlling pills do. Moreover, consuming apple cider vinegar before sleeping lowers fasting blood sugar levels. Scientists have confirmed the fact that regular consumption of apple cider vinegar can considerably improve insulin secretion.

Ways to Consume Apple Cider vinegar for Diabetes

Here are some simple ways of consuming apple cider vinegar:

- Add 1tabespoon of apple cider vinegar to a glass of water and drink twice a day.
- Season sliced cucumbers with 1 tablespoon of apple cider vinegar and eat once a day.
- Mix 1 tablespoon of honey with two tablespoons of apple cider vinegar. Consume this mixture before breakfast.
- Mix 1 tablespoon of love oil, mustard and apple cider vinegar together and use this mixture as a dressing.
- Consume 1 tablespoon of apple cider vinegar twice a day with lemonade or iced tea.
- Dissolve 1 tablespoon of honey and apple in a glass of water and consume it twice a day.

- Dissolve 1 tablespoon of apple cider vinegar and few drops of Stevia in 8 oz. water. Drink it before every meal.

4.7. Apple Cider Vinegar for Yeast Infection

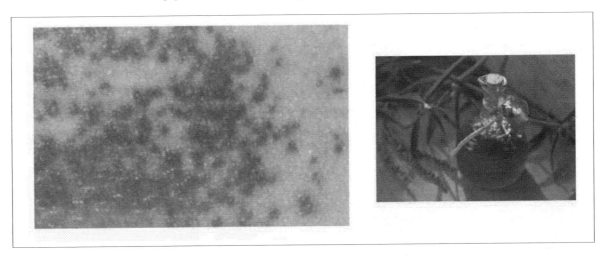

While a number of people rely on over the counter ointments for treating Yeast infection, there are some natural remedies which can permanently cure this fungal infection. One of the most reliable natural remedies for curing yeast infection permanently is apple cider vinegar.

Unlike ointments like Difulcan and Monistat which cure symptoms of the infection and not the cause, apple cider vinegar acts as an anti-fungal agent and kills the fungus. Moreover, apple cider vinegar only fight against harmful bacteria, while pharmaceutical medicines often kill good bacteria too. So, consuming good quality organic apple cider vinegar can permanently cure yeast infection.

How to Use Apple Cider Vinegar for Yeast Infection

Here are some simple ways of using apple cider vinegar for curing yeast infection:

For External Use

External symptoms of yeast infection include itching, rashes and burning of skin. Apple cider vinegar can cure these symptoms. All you have to do is to take hot water apple cider vinegar bath daily. For an apple cider vinegar bath you need to add 2-3 cups of white apple cider vinegar to warm water and soak for 10 minutes. For sever itching, repeat the process twice a day.

For Oral Use

Drinking apple cider vinegar solution daily can help you get rid of the root cause of yeast infection. Apple cider vinegar removes harmful toxins from the body and strengthens the immune system. Moreover, this natural health tonic reduces Candida present inside the body. Although you can easily find apple cider vinegar tablets from a pharmaceutical store, but it is recommended to consume apple cider vinegar in its natural form. Here is a simple way to do so:

- 1 cup water
- Apple cider vinegar, 2-3 tablespoons
- Lemon juice, 2-3 drops

Add lemon juice and apple cider vinegar to a cup of distilled water. Consume this solution twice a day. If you find the taste too strong, you can add 1 teaspoon of honey or maple syrup to the mixture.

For Rinsing

Add 3-4 tablespoons of god quality white apple cider vinegar to warm water. Use the mixture as an anti-bacteria rinsing solution. Apply the mixture twice a day to the infected areas. You can also increase the frequency of usage in order to cure the infection permanently. You can also apply this solution to sensitive areas like vagina.

4.8. Apple Cider Vinegar for Arthritis

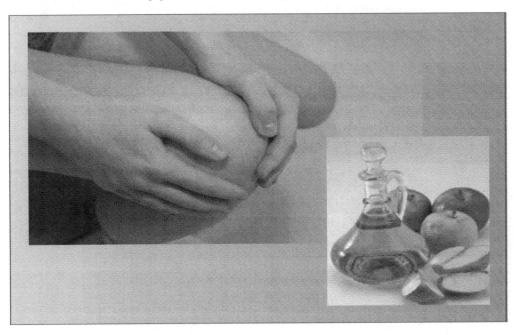

Apple cider vinegar is not only an effective remedy for weight loss, but its daily consumption can also help in regular intake of vitamins, iron and minerals. As the organic tonic is highly rich in magnesium, potassium and phosphorus, it can also be used to cure joint pain and arthritis. Potassium deficiency can also cause joint stiffness, but daily intake of apple cider vinegar reduces the risk of joint problems.

One to overcome mineral deficiencies is to facilitate proper absorption of nutrients into the blood. Apple cider vinegar consists of a number of acids and enzymes which ensure proper functioning of digestive system. Consuming 1 tablespoon of apple cider vinegar before every meal helps in complete absorption of nutrients and accelerating metabolic activities. You can rely on long term therapies and medication to cure arthritis, but apple cider vinegar offers a natural way to cure this joint problem.

Apple Cider Vinegar Cure for Arthritis

Here are two simple ways to make apple cider vinegar tonic for arthritis treatment:

Honey-Vinegar Tonic

1.5 cups of distilled water

Raw honey, 1 teaspoon

White apple cider vinegar, 1 tablespoon

Mix all the ingredients together. Consume the mixture twice a day or before every meal.

Peppermint-Vinegar Tonic

1 cup of distilled water (warm)

Raw honey, 1 tablespoon

Apple cider vinegar, 1 tablespoon

Cinnamon, 1 teaspoon

1 peppermint teabag

Mix all the ingredients together and drink one cup before every meal. Along with facilitating proper potassium consumption, peppermint in the mixture also helps in stabilizing blood pressure and cinnamon helps in controlling blood sugar levels.

4.9. Apple Cider Vinegar for High Cholesterol

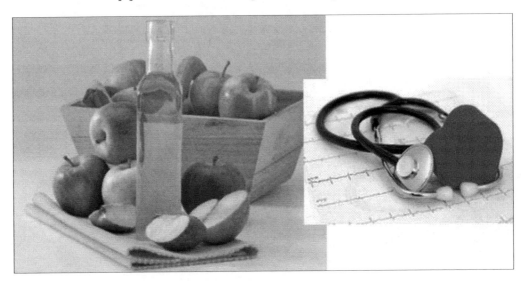

People have been using apple cider vinegar to control cholesterol levels. Recent experimental studies have confirmed the fact that regular intake of apple cider vinegar can help in reducing LDL (harmful cholesterol) while maintaining the HDL levels in the body. Although you can find a number of over the counter drugs for reducing cholesterol, but most of these drugs also reduce HDL which is needed by the body.

How to Consume?

Here are some simple ways of consuming apple cider vinegar on the daily basis:

- Although a number of people find the taste of apple cider vinegar too strong to consume in raw form, taking 2 tablespoons of raw apple cider vinegar can quickly lower cholesterol levels.
- Another way to consume apple cider vinegar is to use it as a salad dressing. Just toss low calorie raw vegetables and fruits together and season them with your favorite apple cider dressing. You can find some amazing dressing recipes in this eBook.
- Add two tablespoons of maple syrup/raw honey and apple cider vinegar to a glass of water and drink it twice a day.
- You can also add 2 tablespoons of apple cider vinegar to a glass of lemonade or iced tea.

4.10. Apple Cider Vinegar for High Blood Pressure

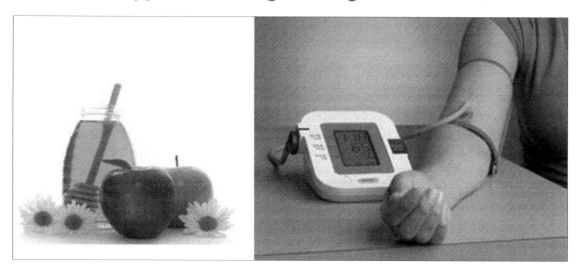

High blood pressure is one of the most common health problems in the world. High blood pressure often leads to stress or nervous breakdown. A number of people rely on prescribed drugs but most of these medicines lower blood pressure by controlling the nervous system.

These medicines are lifetime drugs and there are a number of side effects of these medicines. However, relying on natural remedies for controlling high blood pressure can help you in treating this disease without impacting health. One of the most effective natural remedies for high blood pressure is apple cider vinegar. Apple cider vinegar acts as a health tonic by lowering the LDL levels and reducing the risk of diseases like high blood pressure.

Apple Cider Vinegar with Honey Remedy

Doctors recommend minimum use of salt in order to reduce sodium consumption. But relying on sodium free diet also results in the deficiency of other minerals like potassium. Apple cider vinegar is extremely rich in potassium. All you have to do is take a mixture of 1 tablespoon of apple cider vinegar and raw honey thrice a day or before every meal.

It is recommended to take precautionary measures along with relying on apple cider vinegar for reducing high blood pressure.

Apple Cider Vinegar with Salads

It is very important for high blood pressure patents to avoid oily foods. One of the best ways of doing so is rely on low calorie fresh vegetables and salads. Instead of using salt and pepper to add favor to the salad, use apple cider vinegar dressing for seasoning.

Mixture of vegetables, fruits and apple cider vinegar does not only help in reducing health risks like high blood pressure, but it also provides you a low calorie healthy diet.

Apple Cider Vinegar with Cayenne Pepper

Add 1 teaspoon of cayenne pepper and 1 tablespoon of white apple cider vinegar to a cup of water. Consume the tonic twice a day. It is believed that this is one the most effective natural remedies to cure high blood pressure, as cayenne pepper is known for lowering cholesterol and regulating blood pressure.

5. Uses of Apple Cider Vinegar

Apple cider vinegar is not only known for its countless health benefits, but it can also be used as a beauty care product, anti-septic ointment and what not. Here is a quick look at some of the many uses of apple cider vinegar, which you will be amazed to know.

5.1. Toner

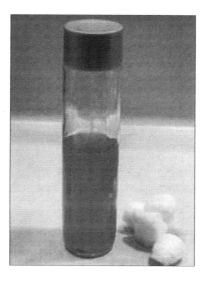

The cleansing action of apple cider vinegar makes it an excellent toner. Apple cider vinegar contains large quantities of acetic, lactic and malic acids which act as skin softeners. Apple cider vinegar keeps the skin healthy by removing dead skin and dust particles. Unlike inorganic skin toners apple cider vinegar helps in maintaining the proper pH of the skin.

Apple Cider Vinegar Toner

You can easily make apple cider vinegar toner at home, by following these simple steps:

- Take ½ cup of White apple cider vinegar and ½ cup of distilled water.
- Mix the ingredients together in a large bowl.
- Take an air tight glass bottle for storing the mixture.
- Pour the mixture in the bottle.
- Shake vigorously.
- Store the toner in a cool and dark place.

Application Directions

- Wash your face with normal face wash.
- Apply the toner with a cotton ball.

- It is recommended using apple cider vinegar skin toner before sleeping.

5.2. Mouth Wash

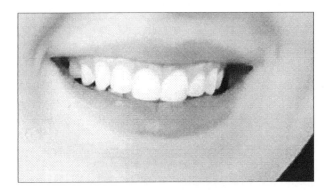

Dentists recommend regular intake of folic acid for healthy and white teeth. Apple cider vinegar contains large quantities of folic acid and thus can be used as a mouthwash. Although the organic acidic tonic can serve the purpose of mouth wash and prevent tooth decay, improper or excessive use of apple cider vinegar can erode the tooth enamel. Therefore it is important to follow a proper formula to use apple cider vinegar as a mouth wash.

Apple Cider Vinegar Mouth Wash

Many toothpastes and mouth wash solutions fail to remove the deposits of tartar, but apple cider vinegar can effectively remove food particles and tartar. All you have to is dissolve 1 teaspoon of apple cider vinegar in a glass of water and use it twice a day.

The mouth wash is not only effective in teeth whitening, but it also prevents tooth decay and cavities. You can also add few leaves of mint.

5.3. Face Mask

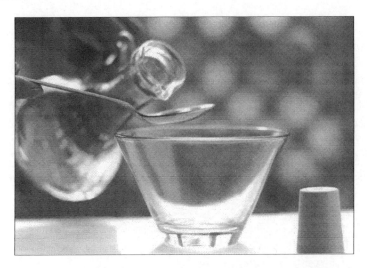

Apple cider can also serve the purpose of a multi-vitamin face mask. This acidic mixture can balance the pH of your skin and keeps it fresh by removing oil and dust deposits. Although apple cider vinegar contains a mixture of weak acids, concentrated vinegar might cause skin burning and itching. Therefore, it is very important to dilute apple coder vinegar before applying it to the face. Moreover, apple cider vinegar also exfoliates dead skin and prevents clogged pores.

Skin requirements vary with the nature of the skin, apple cider vinegar of pH 3 can suit all skin types. Unlike other face masks, apple cider vinegar also has the ability to prevent skin infections, as it is an excellent anti-bacterial solution.

Apple Cider Vinegar Face Mask

Following steps can help you make apple cider vinegar face mask at home:

- Dissolve 1 cup of apple cider vinegar and honey in 2 cups of water.
- Pour the solution in an air tight glass bottle.
- Shake the bottle well.
- Apply the mask for 1-2 hours.
- Wash your face with regular face wash.

5.4. Bath Solution

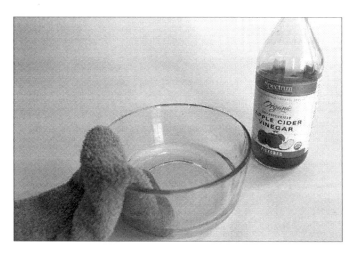

Apple cider vinegar bath solution can cure a number of skin infections and also maintains the pH of the skin. Moreover, warm apple cider vinegar bath can restore the moisture of your skin without making it oily. It is an excellent skin softener and skin cleanser. Moreover, apple cider vinegar can also relief joint pain and cure stiff muscles.

Apple Cider Vinegar Bath Solutions

Here are two simple ways to use apple cider vinegar as a bath solution:

- Take 8 oz. of white apple cider vinegar, 3 cups of kosher salt and few drops of ginger juice. Mix all the ingredients together. Add the mixture to a warm water bath. Soak for 1 hour.

- Dissolve 16 oz. of apple cider vinegar in a hot bath and soak for 1 hour. Take apple cider vinegar bath twice a week for quick results.

5.5. Wart Removal

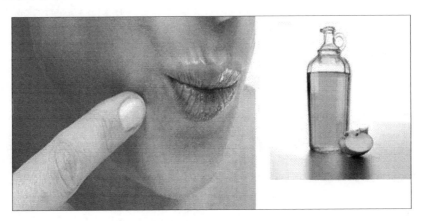

A number of people suffer from warts, which is one of the most common dermatological problems. Although there are a number of ointments and medicines to treat warts, most of these are expensive and have side effects.

Apple cider vinegar is an organic skin toner which can also help in wart removal. Warts are caused when a virus (HPV) enters the body through an open wound or cut. As apple cider vinegar is an anti-septic solution, it not only treats warts but also kills the HPV virus present inside the body.

Wart Removal Remedy

Here is a simple remedy which can help in removing warts painlessly:

- Take a cotton ball and soak it into apple cider vinegar.
- Apply apple cider vinegar to the wart.
- Hold the apple cider vinegar soaked cotton ball in the pace and secure it with a band-aid,
- Peel the band-aid after 24 hours.
- Repeat the same procedure until the wart turns black.

It might take a week for the wart to turn black.

5.6. Veins Treatment

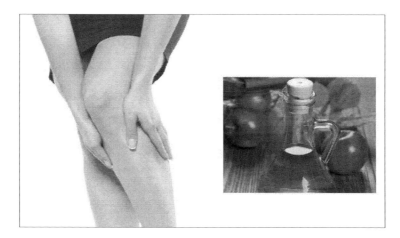

Varicose vein is a painful condition in which veins become twisted and enlarged. There are hundreds of medicines to treat varicose veins, but none of these medicines can fix the problem permanently. Moreover, these medicines are expensive and a person who suffers from varicose veins has to spend a good amount of money on medicines.

However, there are a number of natural remedies which are affordable and can treat varicose veins completely. One of these remedies is apple cider vinegar.

Apple Cider Vinegar Veins Cure

You can cure varicose veins through following methods:

- Take raw apple cider vinegar of good quality. Make sure that the vinegar is not diluted. For quick results choose concentrated apple cider vinegar. Massage varicose veins with apple cider vinegar before going to bed. You can also massage anytime during the day.
- Dissolve two tablespoons of apple cider vinegar in a glass of water. Drink it every day before breakfast. You can add a pinch of maple syrup.

5.7. Deodorant

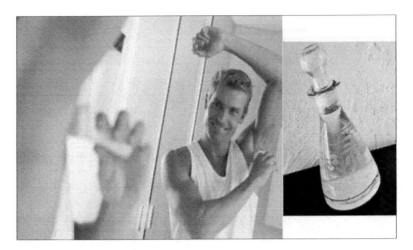

Have you ever wondered how deodorants work? Deodorants clog sweating pores and reduce sweating. As sweating is very important for maintaining the pH of the skin and regulating minerals, clogging of swearing pores can cause several skin infections and problems. Moreover, deodorants contain potentially harmful chemicals which can cause skin cancer. So it is recommended to avoid deodorants and perfumes. However, you can rely on natural products to minimize body odors.

One of the commonly available natural products which can serve the purpose of a deodorant is apple cider vinegar. Add few drops of rose essence to apple cider vinegar to reduce the vinegary smell and apply it to underarms.

5.8. Sun burn Remedy

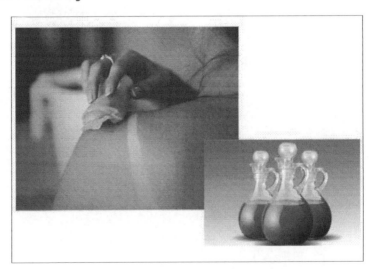

Although sunlight is an excellent source of vitamin D, exposure to sunlight can cause sunburn. Apple cider vinegar can work wonders for restoring skin color and removing sunburn patches. Just add two cups of apple cider vinegar to hot bath and soak for 15-20 minutes.

5.9. Stomach Issues

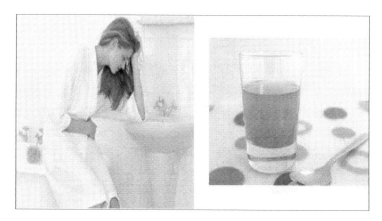

Stomach issues are caused due to abnormal or excessive secretion of stomach acids. Apple cider vinegar contains a mixture of weak acids, which neutralizes the ph of stomach acids and thus cures stomach issues like stomach ache, acid reflux. Just dissolve 2 tablespoons of honey and apple cider vinegar in a glass of water and consume it before every meal. Apple cider vinegar also facilitates proper functioning of digestive system.

5.10. Stuffy Nose

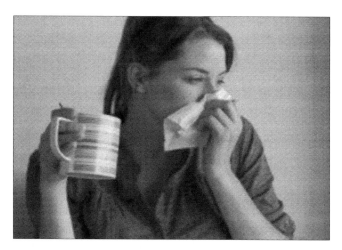

Stuffyy nose is caused due to extreme congestion in nasal and chest cavities. Inhaling apple cider vinegar can help you get rid of stuffy nose within no time. All you have to do is boil apple cider vinegar and inhale the vapors. Apple cider vinegar also fights flu virus.

5.11. Hiccups

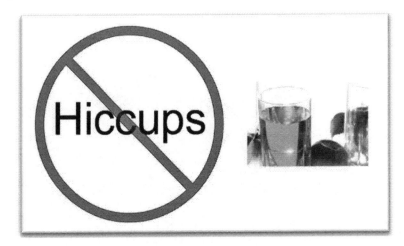

Hiccups are caused due to frequent contraction of diaphragm. Although people mostly rely on home remedies like eating sugar, drinking water or holding breath for hiccups, these remedies are slow. A quick way to stop hiccups is consume 1 tablespoon of concentrated apple cider vinegar. Apple cider vinegar facilitates proper contraction of diaphragm and stops hiccups within minutes.

5.12. Swelling/Sore Throat

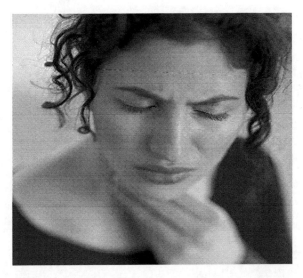

Sore throat is caused due to viral attacks. A number of people rely on antibiotics to cure throat infection, but excessive use of antibiotics can weaken the immune system. However, relying on natural remedies like apple cider vinegar can cure sore throat in a healthy way. Apple cider vinegar acts as an anti-bacterial solution and consuming it in raw form can quickly cure throat infection. Consume 1 tablespoon of apple cider vinegar daily or you can also consume it with honey.

5.13. Leg Cramps

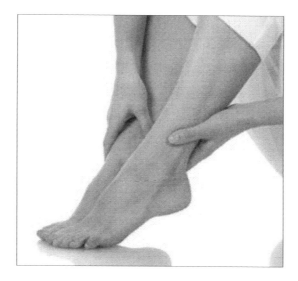

Leg cramps are caused due to abnormal leg muscle contraction. Dehydration and potassium deficiency are two of the prime reasons for leg cramps. For curing dehydration, you should drink 8-10 glasses of water. In order to overcome potassium deficiency, consume apple cider vinegar on daily basis which is an excellent source of potassium. Add two tablespoons of honey and apple cider vinegar to a glass of water and drink it before sleeping.

5.14. Exhaustion

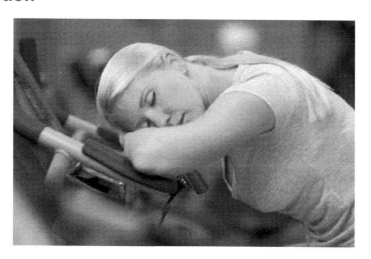

Exhaustion is caused due to improper functioning of adrenal gland. Adrenal secrete hormones which decide human body's response during different situations. However, studies have shown that imbalanced level of blood sugar impact the functioning of adrenal gland. Apple cider vinegar is an organic tonic which helps in maintaining normal blood sugar levels and ensures proper functioning of adrenal gland. Dissolve 2 tablespoons of apple cider vinegar in a glass of water and consume it daily, before breakfast. It will keep you fresh and active.

5.15. Bad Breath

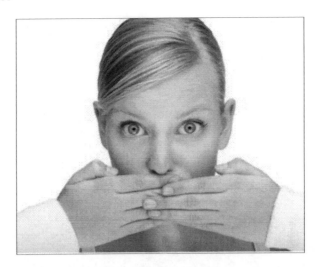

Using apple cider vinegar as a mouth wash not whitens teeth, but also prevents bad breath. Bad breath is caused due to the presence of harmful bacteria in saliva. Apple cider vinegar has an excellent potential to fight against all kinds of harmful bacteria. To make an apple cider vinegar mouth wash, you need to dissolve two tablespoons of pure apple cider vinegar to a glass of water and use the mouth wash twice after brushing your teeth. For long lasting effect you can add few leaves of pepper mint.

5.16. Skin Fungus

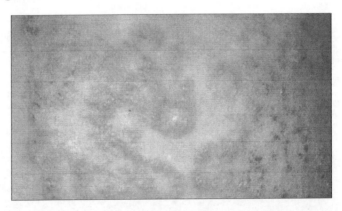

Apple cider vinegar is a homogenous mixture of a number of acids. It is not only an effective health tonic, but also an anti-septic solution. Apple cider vinegar can be used to treat all kinds of skin infections caused by fungus attack. All you have to do is to apply raw apple cider vinegar to the infected area like a lotion. Repeat the procedure twice a day and get rid of skin fungus without relying on expensive ointments.

5.17. Low Blood Pressure

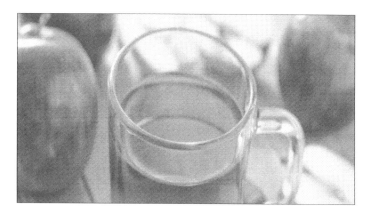

Hypotension or low blood pressure is cause due to deficiency of minerals in the body and dehydration. Apple cider vinegar can effectively help in maintaining the normal blood pressure, as it is highly rich in a number of minerals. Dissolve 2 tablespoons of white apple cider vinegar in a glass of water and consume it twice a day. This remedy can instantly normalize blood pressure. Doctors have confirmed that during pregnancy, consuming apple cider vinegar reduces abrupt variations in blood pressure.

5.18. Age Spots

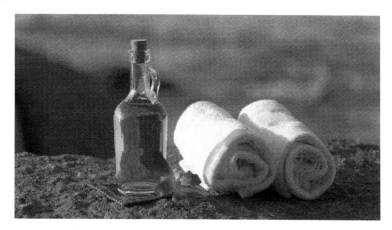

Age spots are cause due to imbalanced pH of the skin. Beauty creams can temporarily cure age spots, but they appear again once you stop using these creams. One way to permanently cure age spots is to apply apple cider vinegar you skin. All you have to do is soak a cotton ball in apple cider vinegar and apply it to age spots. Leave the vinegar on spots for 20 minutes and then wash the area with cold water.

6. Easy Homemade Apple Cider Vinegar Recipes

The best way to consume apple cider vinegar on daily basis is to include it in your daily food intake. Here are some healthy and easy to cook apple cider vinegar recipes which can help in regular consumption of this healthy organic tonic.

6.1. Lunch

Here are some low fat lunch apple cider vinegar recipes which are not only healthy but also quick to prepare:

Apple Cider Vinegar with Fried Chicken and Onion

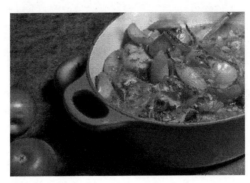

Ingredients

Apple cider vinegar, ¼ cup

Apple cider, 1 cup

2 tart apples

2 onions

Boneless chicken breasts, 1.5 pounds

Chicken broth, 2 cup

Flour, 3 tablespoons

Salt, ½ tablespoon

Olive oil, 1 tablespoon

Fresh rosemary, 1 teaspoon

Directions

Heat olive oil into a pan and add finely chopped onions. Fry onions over medium flame for 15 minutes. Add chopped apples and stir fry with onions for 5 minutes. Remove fried apples and onions from the pan. Coat drained chicken pieces with flour and shallow fry in olive oil. As soon as the chicken turns golden, add apple cider vinegar, apple cider and chicken broth to fried chicken and stir well. Dish out chicken pieces and sprinkle fried apple and onions on the top.

Nutritional Values (Per Serving)

Calories: 264g Carbs: 34g, Fiber: 7g, Protein: 24g, Fat: 6g

Apple Cider Vinegar Roasted Vegetables

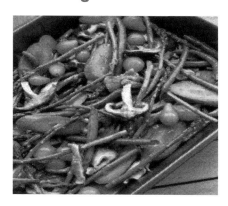

Ingredients

2 Portobello mushrooms

2 carrots

Half purple cabbage

1 onion

Cauliflower, 1 cup

Beans, 1 cup

Broccoli florets, 1.5 cups

Garlic (finely chopped)

Olive oil, 3 tablespoons

Apple cider, 1 cup

Apple cider vinegar, 3 tablespoons

Honey, 1 tablespoon

Directions

Mix apple cider vinegar, cider and honey in a pan and heat over medium flame to blend all the ingredients well. Shallow fry all chopped vegetables together. Toss roasted vegetables in a large bowl and season with apple cider vinegar sauce. Add spices if you want.

Nutritional Values (Per Serving)

Calories: 385.9g Carbs: 80.4g, Fiber: 14.8g, Protein: 8.4g, Fat: 7.8g

6.2. Dinner

You can also add apple cider vinegar to your favorite dinner recipes and convert these dishes into low calorie diet. Here are some must try apple cider vinegar recipes:

Baked Chicken with Apple Cider Vinegar

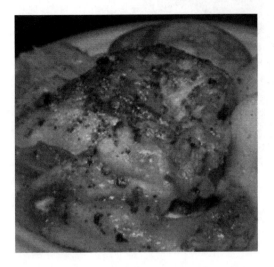

Ingredients

Apple cider vinegar, 1 cup

Boneless chicken, 6 skinless pieces

Garlic salt, 5-6 teaspoons

Directions

Rinse chicken pieces thoroughly. Preheat the oven to 177°C (350°F). Drain the chicken before placing into the oven. Take a 9x13 baking dish and place chicken pieces in it. Coat chicken with apple cider vinegar and sprinkle garlic salt all over the vinegar coated chicken. Place the baking dish into preheated oven and bake for 40 minutes. Enjoy baked chicken with spicy sauces. To add flavor you can also season chicken with chili garlic sauce before baking.

Nutritional Values (Per Serving)

Calories: 680g Carbs: 19g, Fiber: 2, Protein: 48g, Fat: 45g

Apple Cider Vinegar glazed Pork Chops

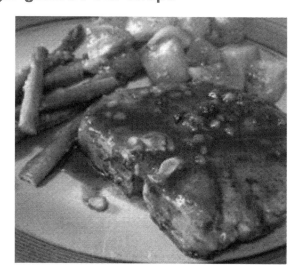

Ingredients

Apple cider vinegar, ¼ cup

Boneless pork chops (center-cut), 6 ounce

Apple cider, 2 cups

Minced garlic, 3 cloves

Salt (to taste)

Black pepper (to taste)

Dijon mustard, 1teaspoon

Rosemary, 1 teaspoon

Oil, 1 tablespoon

Butter, 1 tablespoon

Directions

Start with seasoning chops with pepper and salt. Put butter and oil in a pan and heat then together over medium flame. Shallow fry seasoned chops until browned. It will take 7 to 10 minutes per side. Make sure that chops are tender and juicy. Dish out shallow fried chops and start preparing vinegar sauce. Heat minced garlic for 30 seconds. Pour apple cider vinegar and stir. Add mustard and apple cider to the mixture. Keep stirring the sauce for 5-6 minutes until it is thick and reduced. Finally add rosemary to the sauce and season it with alt and spice to taste. Pour the sauce over chops and coat them uniformly with it.

Nutritional Values (Per Serving)

Calories: 259g Carbs: 19g, Fiber: 2g, Protein: 22g, Fat: 10g

6.3. Drinks

There is no denying the fact that drinking apple cider vinegar on regular basis is very beneficial for health but a number of people don't like the taste of apple cider vinegar. Here are some apple cider drinks which are not only healthy but also delicious.

Apple Cider Vinegar Detox

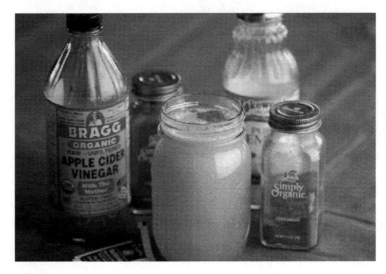

Ingredients

Distilled water, 2 cups

Lemon juice, 2 tablespoons

Stevia powder, 1 packet

Apple cider vinegar, 2 tablespoons

Cinnamon, 1 teaspoon

Cayenne pepper, 1 tablespoon (optional)

Directions

Heat distilled water for 2-3 minutes over medium flame. Add all the ingredients and stir well. Allow the mixture to cool down. Consume it twice a day.

Nutritional Values (Per Serving)

Calories: 6g Carbs: 0g, Fiber: 0g, Protein: 0g, Fat: 0g

Apple Cider Vinegar Cocktail

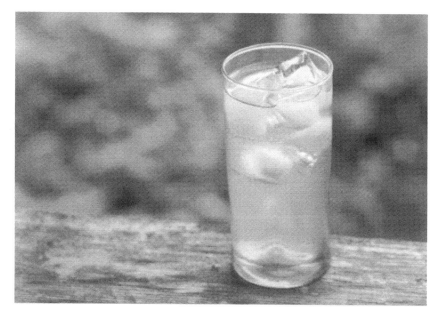

Ingredients

Apple Cider Vinegar (white preferably), 2 teaspoons

Distilled water, 1 cup

Molasses, 1 teaspoon

1 lemon

Directions

Dissolve molasses into distilled water. Add apple cider vinegar and lemon juice to the mixture. Add sugar if desired. Drink the low calorie apple cider cocktail thrice a day.

Nutritional Values (Per Serving)

Calories: 21g Carbs: 5.5g, Fiber: 0g, Protein: 0g, Fat: 0g

6.4. Salads

The best way to consume apple cider vinegar in a healthy way is to add this healthy tonic to vegetable and fruit salads. Raw fruit and vegetable salads can help you in cutting down fat by reducing daily calorie intake and apple cider vinegar accelerates the process of weight loss. Here are some healthy apple cider vinegar salad recipes which can serve the purpose of fat free lunch/dinner.

Apple Cider Vinegar Harvest Salad

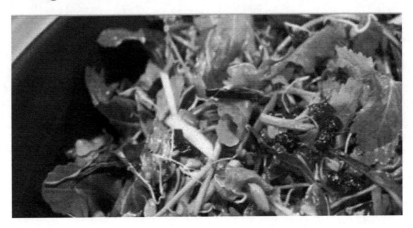

Ingredients

Apple cider vinegar, ½ cup

Dandelion leaves, 2 bunches

1 unpeeled apple (green or red)

Honey, ½ cup (you can also use maple syrup instead of honey)

1 quarter thinly sliced red cabbage

Dijon mustard, 1 tablespoon

Sprouts, 2 handfuls

Olive oil, 1 cup

Arugula leaves, 2 handfuls

Directions

Shred the unpeeled apple to matchstick size. Pour honey, olive oil, mustard and apple cider vinegar in a jar and mix the together. You can also whisk these ingredients in a bowl if you want. Toss all the remaining ingredients in a large bowl. Use the apple cider vinegar dressing to season the salad. Use as much dressing as you want and store the rest in refrigerator. The dressing can stay good for months.

Nutritional Values (Per Serving)

Calories: 160g Carbs: 11g, Fiber: 0g, Protein: 2g, Fat: 12g

Apple Cider Vinegar Mushroom Salad

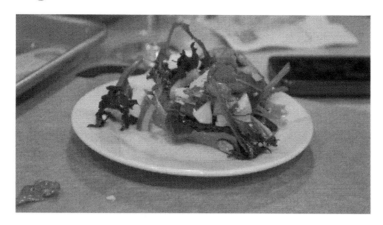

Ingredients

Apple Cider Vinegar, 2 tablespoons

1/ cucumber, sliced

1 tomato, sliced

2 mushrooms

Garlic powder, 1 teaspoon

Black pepper, ¼ teaspoon

Basil, ¼ teaspoon

Salt, ¼ teaspoon

Distilled water, 2 tablespoons

Directions

Toss sliced mushrooms, tomato and cucumber together in a large bowl. Pour apple cider vinegar in another small bowl and add water, salt, pepper and garlic powder to it. Mix all the ingredients well and season the raw vegetables with the apple cider vinegar mixture. As there is no oil used in the recipe, it is an extremely low calorie salad. To add flavor, you can add a pinch of honey or maple syrup.

Nutritional Values (Per Serving)

Calories: 51g Carbs: 12.1g, Fiber: 0g, Protein: 2.8g, Fat: 0.4g

6.5. Desserts

Apple cider vinegar is not only used for seasoning, but it can also give a unique taste to desserts. Here are some easy to cook recipes of apple cider vinegar desserts, you must try.

Apple Cider Vinegar Sponge Cake

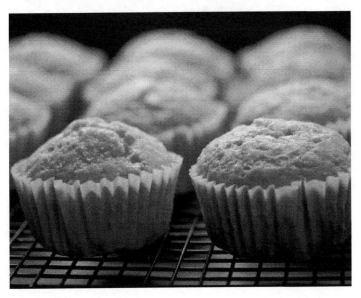

Ingredients

Apple cider vinegar, 1 teaspoon

Soymilk, 1.5 cups

Baking powder, 2 teaspoons

Flour, 2 cups

Baking soda, 1 teaspoon

Cornstarch, 1 tablespoon

Oil, ¼ cup

Salt, ½ teaspoon

Vanilla Extract, 1 teaspoon

Almond Extract (optional), 1 teaspoon

Directions

Mix apple cider vinegar with soymilk. Preheat the oven to 375° F. Add oil to the mixture and whisk well. Combine sugar, cornstarch, flour, salt, baking soda and baking powder together in a large bowl and mix well. Add soymilk and vinegar blend to the mixture and fold. Keeping folding the mixture until combined. Take cupcake molds and fill them with batter. As the batter expands on baking so dun fill the molds fully. Put the molds on preheated oven and bake for 25 minutes. Remove from oven and allow cooling. Decorate with desired topping or chocolate sprinkles.

Nutritional Values (Per Serving)

Calories: 300g Carbs: 50g, Fiber: 1g, Protein: 20g, Fat: 0.4g

Apple Cider Vinegar Ice Pops

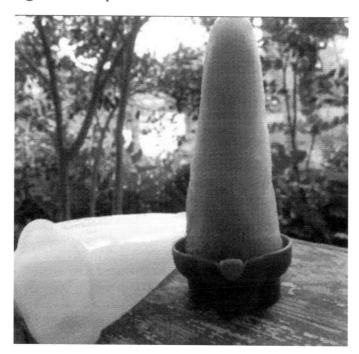

Ingredients

Apple cider vinegar, 4 teaspoons

Apple juice, 4 cups

Sugar, ½ cup

1 cinnamon stick

Vanilla extract, ¼ teaspoon

Directions

Combine water, apple juice and sugar in a sauce pan and heat the mixture to boil. Keep stirring for 25 minutes. Allow the mixture to cool down and add apple cider vinegar and vanilla extract to the mixture. Pour the blend into molds and freeze overnight.

Nutritional Values (Per Serving)

Calories: 72g Carbs: 18g, Fiber: 0g, Protein: 0g, Fat: 0g

6.6. Dips and dressings

Apple Cider Vinegar Strawberry Dressing

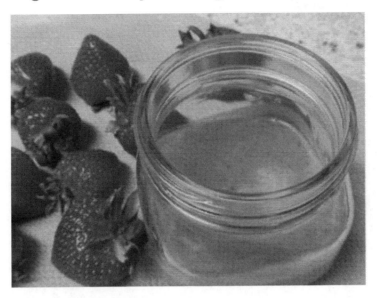

Ingredients

Good quality white apple cider vinegar, 2 tablespoons

Strawberries, 1.5 cups

Olive oil, 2 tablespoons

Turvia (or sugar), 2 cups

Directions

Slice strawberries into small pieces. Blend all the ingredients together. Store the dressing in a glass or plastic jar and refrigerate. You can use the dressing as dessert toping.

Nutritional Values (Per Serving)

Calories: 152.4g Carbs: 10.6g, Fiber: 2.5g, Protein: 0.6g, Fat: 14.4g

Apple Cider Vinegar Honey Dressing

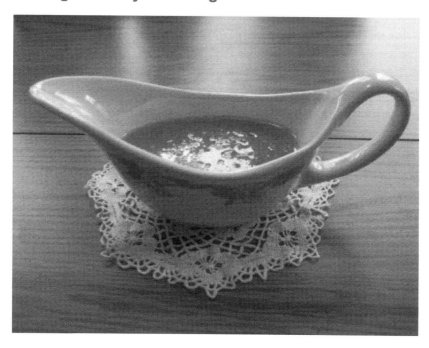

Ingredients

Apple cider vinegar, ¼ cup

Salt, 1.5 teaspoons

Pepper, ¼ teaspoon

Olive oil, 1 cup

Honey, 2 tablespoons

Water, 2 tablespoons

Directions

Combine all the ingredients together and blend well. Keep the mixture in an air tight jar and refrigerate. The dressing can stay good for months if stored properly. Use the low calorie and healthy dressing in salads and desserts.

Nutritional Values (Per Serving)

Calories: 262g Carbs: 5.9g, Fiber: 0g, Protein: 0g, Fat: 27g

Final Words

Apple cider vinegar is not only used for cooking, but it also serves the purpose of an organic health tonic. This report includes a number of ways through which apple cider vinegar can cure chronic diseases. Moreover, the eBook also contains some other uses of apple cider vinegar which you will be amazed to know. You can also find some amazing lunch, dinner, and dessert recipes in this eBook, which can facilitate adequate apple cider vinegar consumption on daily basis.

Try these apple cider remedies and recipes and enjoy countless health benefits!

Made in the USA
Middletown, DE
26 August 2019